The Diabetes Defense: Practical Tips and Hacks to Shut Down Your Genetic Risk

The Diabetes Defense: Practical Tips and Hacks to Shut Down Your Genetic Risk

Copyright © 2024 by **Omolola Habib**

Table of Content

INTRODUCTION 5

CHAPTER 1: DECODING YOUR GENETIC RISK 7

What Genes Have to Do With Diabetes 7

Strengths and Weaknesses of Genetic Testing 7

Inherited Odds Aren't Destiny 8

CHAPTER 1: DECODING YOUR GENETIC RISK 9

Common Genetic Markers and Variants 9

Strengths and Limitations of Genetic Testing 11

Putting Your Genetic Risk in Perspective 12

Chapter 1 Takeaways: Your DNA is Not Your Destiny 13

CHAPTER 2: DIET AND LIFESTYLE STRATEGIES FOR DEFENSE 16

Evidence-Based Nutrition Tips to Improve Insulin Sensitivity 17

Simple Substitutes to Remove Sugar Traps From Your Diet 18

Realistic Ways to Boost Daily Physical Activity 19

Science-Backed Stress Management Techniques 20

Importance of Sleep for Metabolism and Blood Sugar Control 22

Chapter 2 Takeaways: Your Lifestyle Overpowers Genes 23

CHAPTER 3: DODGING PREDIABETES 25

Criteria for Prediabetes and Early Warning Signs 26

Gradual Progression to Full-Blown Diabetes ... 27

Benefits of Catching Prediabetes Early & Room for Improvement ... 28

Specific Tactics to Reverse Prediabetes Trajectory ... 30

Chapter 3 Takeaways: Destiny is in Your Hands ... 31

CHAPTER 4: SHIELDING YOUR LONG-TERM HEALTH ... 33

Relationship Between Diabetes and Various Complications ... 34

Protecting Your Heart, Blood Vessels, Eyes, Kidneys and Nerves ... 35

Living Well Through Ongoing Management of Biomarkers ... 36

Chapter 4 Takeaways: Where There's Life, There's Hope ... 37

CONCLUSION: NOW GO DEFEND YOUR DESTINY! ... 40

Key Takeaways ... 40

Ongoing Resources ... 41

Final Words: Go Live Vibrantly Now! ... 42

ABOUT THE AUTHOR ... 43

Introduction

The rates of diabetes have been steadily increasing to the point that we are now experiencing a worldwide epidemic. According to the latest statistics from the CDC, over 34 million Americans have diabetes, with approximately 1.5 million new cases diagnosed every year. Given this trajectory, healthcare experts warn that 1 in 3 American adults could develop diabetes in their lifetime if current trends continue.

So why should this concern you? Diabetes significantly raises the risk of numerous disabling and life-threatening health complications, from heart disease and stroke to kidney failure, vision loss and amputation of toes or feet. It also reduces overall quality of life while requiring constant medical treatment and monitoring. Prediabetes frequently leads to type 2 diabetes as well, so this metabolic condition demands attention too. Clearly, diabetes and prediabetes have become major public health challenges.

On an encouraging note, getting diabetes does not have to be an inevitable consequence of aging or genetics. Researchers now understand how insulin resistance develops over time, setting the stage for rising blood sugar levels. Key risk factors under your control include excess weight, especially abdominal fat. Inactivity and loss of muscle mass also reduce the body's ability to respond to insulin and use blood glucose properly. Age, family history and ethnicity can raise risk further, but are not necessarily destiny.

The good news is that numerous large studies on diabetes prevention conclusively show that people can significantly reduce their risk through lifestyle changes. Eating more whole, high fiber carbs while cutting back on meat, unhealthy fats and sugary foods has been proven to increase insulin sensitivity. Regular exercise, stress reduction techniques and adequate sleep also uniquely improve insulin resistance and related biomarkers. Even if genetic risk factors exist, you absolutely have power to "shut down" their impact through daily habits and choices that keep cells responsive to insulin.

In this book, you'll learn practical evidence-based strategies for understanding prediabetes, reducing progression risks and ultimately dodging a type 2 diabetes diagnosis. I'll translate the latest scientific findings on everything from nutrition to fitness to genetics into clear advice anyone can start applying today. You'll come away both informed and empowered to implement a personalized diabetes defense plan, regardless of your starting risk. Remember, it's never too late or too early to take control of your health. Let's get started!

Chapter 1: Decoding Your Genetic Risk

You've probably heard that diabetes runs in families or that certain ethnic groups have higher odds of developing it. So you may be wondering just how much of a role your genes actually play versus lifestyle factors you can control. Here's your plain-language guide to understanding how genetics influence diabetes without getting overwhelmed by the science or feeling like your fate is predetermined!

What Genes Have to Do With Diabetes

Type 2 diabetes is what scientists call a "complex disease," meaning both genetic and environmental factors are at play in causing it. Your DNA provides a basic blueprint that makes developing insulin resistance and high blood sugar more or less likely, but your daily habits and exposures determine how and when those tendencies manifest. Think of genetics loading the gun when it comes to diabetes risk, but your lifestyle pulling the trigger.

Researchers so far have identified over 400 gene variants associated with altered diabetes risk of some kind. Two of the most well-studied are TCF7L2 and PPARG. The first impairs insulin production by the pancreas while the second affects fat cell function. Having these or similar variants is definitely linked to higher odds of becoming diabetic. But again, that doesn't make getting diabetes inevitable or untreatable through healthy daily choices.

Strengths and Weaknesses of Genetic Testing

Given the explosion of direct-to-consumer DNA tests from companies like 23andMe, curiosity about what your personal genetics say about diabetes risk is understandable! When ordered online or through a doctor, these cheek swab kits can indeed pinpoint whether you have any known variant genes.

However, viewing these results in proper context is crucial. First off, the presence of markers does not communicate at what age diabetes may develop or how serious your case could become with poor lifestyle habits over time. Genetic testing also can't yet account for every possible gene-environment interaction, so risks could still be over or underestimated for any one individual.

That said, genetic insight can motivate positive behavior changes and more vigilant screenings for early signs of insulin resistance. In that sense, testing represents one more tool for empowering patients. I help patients every day translate genetic data into concrete prevention strategies personalized to their risks and needs.

Inherited Odds Aren't Destiny

No matter what your ethnic background or family experience with diabetes, don't view inheriting some genetic risk factors as destiny you can't escape. Not everyone with variant genes becomes diabetic. Their impacts clearly interact with diet, activity levels, weight management and other controllable factors starting even in childhood.

While genetics insight can be useful, quickly moving into problem-solving mode around lifestyle changes offers the most power to overcome inherited odds. Later chapters will show exactly how to embark upon that diabetes defense action plan!

Chapter 1: Decoding Your Genetic Risk

Chances are you've wondered about the role genetics play when it comes to diabetes. If the disease runs strongly in your family, you may feel a diagnosis is inevitable no matter what preventive steps you might take. Or awareness of increased type 2 diabetes prevalence within your ethnic community may have you feeling resigned to the same fate. I deeply empathize with those sentiments. Yet the good news is that while biology influences risk, it does not rigidly determine your destiny.

In this chapter, I'll translate the latest scientific insights about diabetes's hereditary factors into plain language so you can understand how genes interact with environment and lifestyle. My goal is to leave you feeling knowledgeable, hopeful and empowered—not anxious or defeated. You'll gain practical, personalized strategies based on your genetic risk profile to counteract any susceptibilities while best protecting future health.

I'll also candidly discuss limitations, contradictions and uncertainties inherent to this emerging field of diabetes genetics so you can evaluate direct-to-consumer tests and screening options from an informed perspective. My commitment extends beyond simply presenting research to helping you apply genetic discoveries in your daily life to maximum effect. Are you ready to decode your diabetes genetic forecast? Let's get started!

Common Genetic Markers and Variants

As we dive deeper, understanding key terminology will help clarify how scientists associate certain gene mutations and single nucleotide polymorphisms (SNPs pronounced "snips") with altered diabetes risk. Don't let the science-y words intimidate you though! I'll be sure to translate concepts into simple takeaways you can actually use.

Mutations

Let's start with mutations – permanent changes within critical gene sequences involved in insulin production, glucose transport, fat cell function and more. Several known mutations stand out:

HNF1A & HNF4A: These rare inherited defects limit insulin output by the pancreas over time. Spotting them early allows quicker treatment before diabetes fully develops.

WFS1: Faulty versions negatively impact insulin secretion and increase stress hormone release. This one ties directly to Wolfram Syndrome featuring vision issues and diabetes.

POMC: When defective, appetite regulation goes haywire, driving obesity and related metabolic disruption. Weight management becomes much more challenging.

SNPs

Now onto SNPs - subtle one letter DNA typos scattered throughout the genomes of all humans. GWAS studies compare SNPs in thousands of people with and without particular diseases to pinpoint risk patterns. For diabetes, 23andMe and other consumer DNA tests screen for a dozen or more SNP variants linked to likelihood of insulin resistance.

Ones tied to blood sugar impairment include:

IRS1: Interferes with insulin signaling, especially in obese women and those of Asian descent.

TCF7L2: Hinders insulin production by pancreatic beta cells so less gets released.

KCNQ1: Impacts how insulin is transported and regulated at the cellular level over time.

The key reminder is that few SNPs alone directly cause diabetes, but certain genotypes do moderately tune up or down your overall genetic susceptibility.

Strengths and Limitations of Genetic Testing

With genetic testing now accessible directly to consumers through health companies like 23andMe, you may be wondering whether peeking into your DNA crystal ball for diabetes risk clues is worthwhile. Let's weigh some pros and cons so you can decide if learning your genotype empowers or overwhelms!

Potential Benefits

- Creates motivation for protective lifestyle changes and adherence

- Allows early monitoring to catch ascending blood sugar trends

- Screens for rare monogenic mutations to guide treatment

- Provides risk clarity for family members to test or take precautions

- Furthers diabetes research through shared genetic database

Drawbacks and Nuances

- Only partially explains individual's absolute diabetes risk

- Likelihood estimates for SNPs apply to larger populations

- Environment and genes interact in unpredictable ways

- Limited risk attribution for ethnic minorities

- Minimal insight on disease progression timeline

- Psychological stress from sense of helplessness

As with most complex chronic diseases, making personal health decisions based on diabetes genetic test results requires thoughtfulness. I guide my patients through that critical appraisal process so they feel empowered, not overwhelmed.

Here's my suggested mindset regardless of your genetic risk factors: let testing inform and motivate preventive behaviors without it feeling like an inescapable life sentence. After all, daily lifestyle choices wield incredible influence over how weakly or strongly those genes get expressed. Our DNA provides insight, but we still very much control our destiny!

Putting Your Genetic Risk in Perspective

Getting genetic testing results in hand may have left you discouraged or filled with dread about an inevitable diabetes conclusion. Or family history alone may have you bracing for a potential diagnosis even before directly peering into your DNA. Wherever you are starting from, keeping risk realities in perspective is essential so you channel feelings constructively without fatalism dragging you down.

Chapter 1 Takeaways: Your DNA is Not Your Destiny

As we close this chapter exploring the nuances of how genetics relate to diabetes risk, I want to highlight a few key points to empower you on your prevention journey:

1. Genes only load the gun - lifestyle pulls the trigger. While DNA may increase susceptibility, daily habits and environment determine if and how strongly those tendencies manifest. Regular activity, plant-focused diets and other controllable choices, reliably slash diabetes odds by up to 80% even with strong family history.

2. Diabetes genetic risk exists on a continuum. Inheriting certain subtle SNPs or even rarer mutations does not rigidly sentence you to metabolic disruption or high blood sugar over time. Pay attention to lifestyle risk factors within your control rather than obsessing over fixed markers you can't change.

3. Genetic insight supports early screening/detection. If testing does reveal elevated genetic odds, view it as helpful information to motivate monitoring insulin, glucose and inflammation biomarkers so you can respond promptly to signals needing addressed through nutrition, fitness or stress relief tweaks.

4. Probability is not destiny. Testing offers clues about vulnerability based on broad statistics and inheritance patterns – not infallible predictions about any one person's future. Relatives share genes but not necessarily other environment/behavior variables converging to enable disease.

5. All bodies have relative strengths and weaknesses. Rather than scare or defeat you, let your genetic results guide you to focus preventive efforts where your biology most needs support. Then dial up lifestyle buffers best counterbalancing those susceptibilities.

I hope this crash course on the real-life implications of diabetes genetic risk empowers you on the path ahead! Remember, your DNA provides insights to work with, not limitations to work against. Onward!

A few clarifying reminders to help genetics speak rather than shout at you:

- Genetic risk for type 2 diabetes manifests as a spectrum - not everyone with susceptibilities develops disease. Lifestyle choices make a profound difference.

- Your DNA provides information about biological vulnerability based on broad population statistics - it is not an infallible individual fortune teller.

- Relatives share genes but not necessarily living environments and habits that converge to trigger disease. Their diabetes does not guarantee your fate.

- Ethnicity-based risks cite group tendencies only - considerable variation amongst individuals exists. Not every member of high-risk populations becomes diabetic.

- While useful, genetic markers reveal probability not certainty. Most common diabetes gene variants only slightly nudge overall risk up or down.

In a world shouting genetic determinism, remembering your lifestyle power and agency matters most. Even with a double dose of "risk genes," daily movement, plant-based diets, managed stress and other controllable behaviors reliably slash diabetes likelihood by half or more. Our manifesting destiny combines gene influences with self-directed environmental inputs - so make sure yours point favorably in a healthy direction!

Chapter 2: Diet and Lifestyle Strategies for Defense

In the last chapter, we confronted the reality that genes do play a role in diabetes risk by tuning biological factors up or down for each unique individual. I emphasized, however, that DNA only loads the gun when it comes to your odds of developing prediabetes or type 2 diabetes. Daily lifestyle behaviors and environment ultimately determine if and how strongly genetic susceptibilities get expressed.

The empowering news is that multiple major studies on thousands of participants conclusively demonstrate that even with strong family histories, people can dramatically reduce their likelihood of impaired insulin/glucose metabolism through controllable lifestyle strategies. We're talking, cutting risk factors almost in half with straightforward, sustainable habit changes!

In this chapter, I'll distill reams of nutrition and fitness research into clear action steps so you can start implementing an integrated diabetes defense plan. You'll discover how simple food swaps, stress relief techniques, activity additions and sleep habit tweaks make it remarkably easy to upregulate genes promoting healthy blood sugar balance while muting risk-elevating genetic influences happening behind the scenes.

My approach focuses on establishing easy, sustainable healthy rituals rather than demanding quick fixes or perfection. You'll receive balanced lifestyle prescriptions tailored to your unique needs and risk profile. Best of all, I'll share insider tips so adopting new diabetes-defying habits feels exciting rather than overwhelming! The journey of a thousand miles begins with simple steps forward – let's start marching together, shall we?

Evidence-Based Nutrition Tips to Improve Insulin Sensitivity

When it comes to defending your body against diabetes, dietary upgrades make up the front line of lifestyle strategies shown to dramatically reduce risk markers even in the face of genetic predispositions. Supporting healthy insulin sensitivity starts with what you choose to put on your plate!

While specialized diets like intermittent fasting, low-carb plans or the Mediterranean approach each offer perks, I find focusing first on overall eating quality and biodiversity reaps big benefits for stabilizing blood sugar trends. From that balanced foundation, you can then personalize with nutritional tactics tailored to your family history, metabolic test results and body type.

Here are sustainable, flexible real-food diet upgrades I recommend clients build into daily routines for optimizing insulin response and related fat-storage hormones impacted heavily by genetic susceptibilities:

Emphasize Plants & Minimize Process: Focus on getting 20-30 grams of fiber from vegetables, fruits, beans/legumes, whole grains and nuts/seeds daily. Limit human-made packaged items with long ingredient lists.

Balance Blood Sugar Impact: Pair carbs from fruits, whole grains and starchy veggies with protein, fat or vinegar to blunt blood sugar spikes. Think apple slices with nut butter!

Hydrate Wisely: Drink ample water and unsweetened beverages instead of sugary liquids that augment insulin demands. Herbal teas provide antioxidants without spiking insulin like coffee.

Time Meals Mindfully: Avoid long periods without eating during day and lengthy 12+ hour overnight fasts that deregulate hunger-regulating hormones related to insulin.

No need to radically overhaul everything instantly – just regularly swap in upgrades! Over time, these evidence-backed eating strategies compound to deliver huge dividends for your diabetes defense plan!

Simple Substitutes to Remove Sugar Traps From Your Diet

When aiming to stabilize blood sugar trends and insulin needs in preparation for strategic nutrition upgrades, an easy first step involves replacing unnecessary sugar sources sabotaging your diabetes defense efforts. Outright banning sweets rarely works long-term, so I guide clients to start by swapping out stealthy sugars lurking where you may not realize. Before you know it, your palate adapts to prefer natural sweetness!

Here are simple, painless sugar substitute ideas to try:

Yogurt: Rather than fruit-on-the bottom or low-fat sweetened varieties, opt for plain whole milk Greek yogurt. Mix in your own berries and nuts or seeds for fiber and healthy fats to balance sugar response.

Salad Dressings: Skip high fructose corn syrup-laden brands in favor of olive oil and vinegar combos you control. Splash balsamic or real lemon juice over greens instead of dumping on candied dressing that spikes blood sugar.

Sauces & Condiments: Set aside tropical fruit jams, honey mustard and teriyaki in exchange for versatile vinaigrettes, chimichurri sauce or unsweetened BBQ made with diabetes-friendly ingredients you recognize.

Overnight Oats: Trade pre-flavored instant packets for plain rolled or steel-cut oats cooked stovetop then chilled overnight with nuts, seeds and unsweetened almond milk. Adjust taste as needed rather than relying on syrupy mixes.

Box Mix Desserts: Say no to chemicals and added sugars in puddings and cake mixes by whipping up chia pudding, homemade protein bars or fruit-sweetened squares using wholesome ingredients.

Nut Butters: Skip candy-filled peanut butter spreads in favor of DIY nutty blends made simply from nuts/seeds blended to desired creaminess. Then control added mix-ins like unsweetened cocoa or cinnamon.

Remember, gradual small upgrades lead to sustainable change over time! Keep substitutions simple at first while your tastebuds adapt to enjoy food more naturally.

Realistic Ways to Boost Daily Physical Activity

Beyond proper nutrition, ensuring regular movement builds and maintains lean muscle mass essentially creates an internal armor protecting you from expressing diabetes genetic risk factors to their full potential. But endless hours of boring cardio are NOT required!

I guide my clients toward sustainable activity habits providing all-day blood sugar stabilizing effects without demanding sweaty exhaustion or hour counts impossible to tackle between family, career and life demands. Follow these tips for diabetic-defying movement:

Walk More: Aim for 7,000-10,000 daily steps tracked via fitness wearable. Even steady leisurely strolling makes a massive difference vs prolonged sitting and sedentary time.

Try Interval Training: Just 2-3 short sessions weekly alternating intense bursts with recovery translates to enhanced insulin sensitivity and cardio endurance to balance energy.

Incorporate Strength Training: Weight lifting, resistance bands and other muscle-building workouts prompt your body to absorb blood glucose for energy while improving insulin receptor response.

Sit Less: Break up prolonged immobile periods by standing during commercial breaks, using a treadmill desk, taking midday movement breaks. Sitting sabotages hormones.

Just Get Moving: Rather than forcing rigid regimes, focus on enjoying sustainable activity you can maintain lifelong. Gardening, dancing, playing with kids and other movement you barely notice as "exercise" all contributes!

Boosting everyday movement through enjoyable activities creates positive momentum while preventing the blood sugar surges and hormonal shifts that enable diabetes risk genes. The key is consistency, not intensity. Small steps forward make the biggest difference over time!

Science-Backed Stress Management Techniques

You may be surprised to learn unrelenting stress directly antagonizes healthy blood sugar balance by over-activating cortisol, glucagon and other hormones that release stored glucose into the bloodstream. Left unmanaged over years, this rollercoastering of insulin needs puts tremendous strain on your metabolism. That's why proactively building stress resilience bolsters your diabetes defenses even if genetic risk exists.

Thankfully, easy evidence-based relaxation practices begin taming hot-wired neurological pathways in as little as 60-90 seconds daily! Here are techniques I teach clients that research confirms lower biomarkers for insulin resistance and inflammation:

Mindful Breathing: Quiet the mind's stress triggers and cortisol release through 5-10 minutes steadily inhaling and exhaling while focusing only on the present breath. Apps provide guided sessions.

Gratitude Journaling: Refocus the brain away from worry loops toward appreciation by regularly jotting a quick list of current blessings and silver linings. This habit neurologically shifts mood.

Yoga, Tai Chi or Qigong: Gentle flowing sequences harmonize mind, body and spirit while reducing inflammatory stress hormones and stimulating insulin production and receptor sites.

Laugh Out Loud: Make time for comedy breaks watching silly pet videos and seeking humor. Laughter's physical response releases tension while boosting circulation and blood sugar processing.

Hug Loved Ones: Research confirms affectionate contact with other humans calms the nervous system, oxytocin levels and emotional eating urges that can spike blood sugar.

Unplug Frequently: Allow your mind to fully rest without constant digital input so parasympathetic relaxation becomes your body's default mode. Limit devices at night.

Remember, lifelong stress resilience minimizes how strongly adverse genetic variables get expressed. But lifelong doesn't have to start today – just practice 60-90 seconds of go-to stress relief rituals during each part of your day!

Importance of Sleep for Metabolism and Blood Sugar Control

You have likely heard that adequate shut-eye keeps immunity strong, maintains cognitive sharpness and stabilizes moods. But did you know sufficient high-quality sleep also provides powerful protection against developing insulin resistance and diabetes? Research confirms that along with nutrition and activity, ample restorative nightly downtime makes up a third pillar for keeping biomarkers balanced and risk factors in check.

Unfortunately, between work worries, digital distraction, family demands and health issues, many adults today face chronic sleep deprivation. Over years, the compound impact destabilizes hormones directing appetite, weight management and glucose metabolism in directions that silently enable diabetes risk genetics.

But the fantastic news is that relatively quick sleep habit changes reliably reverse metabolic disruption linked to genetic variables! Follow these tips:

Stick to routines: Try to turn lights off and wake up at consistent times to anchor natural circadian rhythms directing hormone fluctuations.

Limit blue light exposure: Dim devices and screens emitting melatonin-disrupting blue wavelengths for 1-2 hours before bedtime to ease falling and staying asleep.

Upgrade your sleep sanctuary: Invest in blackout curtains, comfy bedding and an eye mask/ear plugs to ensure your bedroom promotes deep 8 hour sleep nightly.

Relax through rituals: Practice relaxing meditations, gentle stretches or relax your face/body section by section to cue the mind that it's time for restoration.

Keep cooler: Chilly bedroom temperatures in the 66-69°F range have been shown to induce faster sleep onset, combat night sweats and result in higher-quality sleep.

Remember, awaking feeling genuinely well-rested accumulates benefits over time to keep insulin and glucose markers within optimal ranges! Make sleep a priority regardless of genetic hand you've been dealt.

Chapter 2 Takeaways: Your Lifestyle Overpowers Genes

Congratulations for taking proactive steps to implement a tailored diabetes defense plan regardless of the genetic probabilities you may have inherited! As we wrap up this lengthy chapter full of lifestyle upgrade ideas to get you started, I want to reiterate a few motivational points:

1. Consistency matters more than perfection. Don't let great stand in the way of good enough. Focus first on sticking with any upgrade for 2-3 weeks until it becomes an automatic habit skewing your health destiny daily.

2. All progress is still forward movement. On tough days when willpower wanes, give yourself permission to maintain rather than worrying about perfect adherence. Small steps forward still outweigh standing still.

3. Collaborate with support systems. Enlist household members, friends or social media groups to inspire accountability and encouragement choosing easy wins fitting your real life. This is a lifestyle shift rather than temporary sprint!

4. Prevent overwhelm with pacing. Add just 1-2 new eating, fitness, stress or sleep tweaks per week allowing each to solidify before stacking additional changes. Steady gains avoiding burnout keep you consistently headed the right diabetes-defying direction!

5. Stay focused on controllable actions. When frustration arises, refocus attention on daily choices within your power rather than ruminating over unchangeable diabetes odds defined by your DNA. Progress flows from self-directed rewards-based motivation.

I'll leave you with this final reminder - your genes provide background context, but adopting wise lifestyle habits reflects the foreground focus for preventing disease. Keep placing one foot in front of the other down the positive path of progress rather than letting genetics block your view of possibility! Onward!

Chapter 3: Dodging Prediabetes

If you've been diagnosed with prediabetes or metabolic syndrome, you may feel resigned to eventually developing full-blown type 2 diabetes as part of your genetic destiny. Especially if close relatives struggled to escape that seeming inevitability despite medication compliance. Now facing rising blood sugar trends yourself, frustration and defeatism makes sense.

The fantastic news is that lifestyle upgrades leveraging food as medicine principles can halt and even reverse insulin resistance progression in a significant majority of cases. In fact, the NIH-funded Diabetes Prevention Program study demonstrated that moderate exercise and weight loss of just 5-10% dramatically lowered type 2 diabetes incidence amongst prediabetic individuals by an impressive 58% over 3 years. And that was without expensive medications!

In this chapter, I'll provide clarity around prediabetes testing limitations, evidence-based reversal strategies and early warning signs to monitor even before diagnostic thresholds are met. My aim is to shift perspective from powerlessness in the face of perceived genetic programming to informed action steps dodging deterioration toward diabetes.

Rather than demanding perfection, I guide clients toward sustainable lifestyle solutions optimized to their unique needs. Small consistent changes addressing root causes of metabolic dysfunction accumulate big overtime - like compound interest on your health account! Soon enough, symptoms become less severe, numbers improve, and most importantly, your mindset shifts from hopeless to empowered.

If you or loved ones feel stuck in prediabetes limbo without clear ways forward, get ready for that to change. Grab your notebook and let's get to work unlocking your full vitality potential!

Criteria for Prediabetes and Early Warning Signs

Gaining clarity on how doctors diagnose prediabetes and related markers can empower you to proactively monitor personal risk factors and symptoms long before irreversible disease progression. I guide my patients in understanding key lab tests and recognizing subtle signs often years before official thresholds warrant medications. Early indicators, even if below the prediabetes classification range, provide an opportunity to intervene with lifestyle solutions to divert disease trajectory.

Here's what to know:

Diagnostic Benchmarks

Doctors rely on fasting plasma glucose, oral glucose tolerance tests and hemoglobin A1C blood tests to screen for and track prediabetes severity. Each provide snapshot readings of average blood sugar over recent weeks and months. Crossing the following thresholds prompts prediabetes rather than normal range classification:

- Fasting Plasma Glucose: 100-125 mg/dL

- Oral Glucose Tolerance: 140-199 mg/dL at 2 hour mark

- Hemoglobin A1C: 5.7–6.4%

Subclinical Symptoms

However, research shows insulin dysfunction and glucose impairment begin up to a decade before even slightly high lab ranges are detectable. I coach patients on tuning into common bodily clues and life interference patterns signaling momentum toward prediabetes vulnerability. These include:

- Brain fog/fatigue after meals signaling blood sugar spikes and crashes

- Increasing waist circumference and abdominal weight gain

- Difficulty losing weight despite diet and exercise efforts

- Cravings for sweets and energy crashes signaling imbalanced metabolism

- Rising cholesterol, blood pressure and inflammation lab markers

Catching subtle shifts early allows for nutrition and fitness solutions long before pharmaceutical reliance becomes inevitable.

Gradual Progression to Full-Blown Diabetes

Understanding the step-wise biological progression from prediabetes to eventual type 2 diabetes empowers you to pinpoint exactly where you land on that spectrum. That insight allows for tailored interventions to halt momentum before disease inevitability sets in.

Here's an overview of key milestones as insulin resistance advances:

Insulin Resistance Emergence: The journey begins years before diagnosis as cells gradually lose sensitivity to insulin, forcing the pancreas to overproduce more and more of this hormone to lower blood sugar after meals. This stage usually has no obvious symptoms for 5-10 years.

Prediabetes Onset: Diagnostic thresholds are crossed as fasting glucose nears 100-125 mg/dL, hemoglobin A1c reaches 5.7-6.4% and the pancreas strains to counteract cellular insulin resistance. Modest lifestyle measures can still reverse trajectory for many.

Pancreatic Beta Cell Burnout: Initially, insulin overproduction by the pancreas compensates for decreasing cell sensitivity. But over years, these insulin factories become exhausted and begin slowing production. Blood sugar rises as a result along with overt diabetes symptoms.

Type 2 Diagnosis: Finally, the pancreas cannot keep pace with extreme resistance, fasting blood glucose verifies above 125 mg/dL, glucose spikes grow exaggerated after meals, and symptoms like blurred vision, numbness, recurrent infections and slow healing prompt diagnosis.

The key takeaway is that lifestyle adjustments harness the most power earlier in the disease progression rather than later. I help patients customize plans addressing root causes of their metabolic dysregulation to turn the tide before it's too late. The best diabetes defense is preventing full progression in the first place!

Benefits of Catching Prediabetes Early & Room for Improvement

Given the gradual, step-wise nature of metabolic disease progression, identifying insulin resistance indicators during early subtle stages offers more control over health destiny than waiting until irreparable pancreatic burnout and full-fledged type 2 diabetes manifest. Though early signs feel less scary than a definitive diagnosis, make no mistake - timely lifestyle interventions in the prediabetes zone still provide massive protective effects.

Here's why optimizing diet, activity, sleep and stress management without delay matter:

Halting Momentum

Catching rising glucose and HbA1c trends early allows for nutrition and movement adjustments preventing further deterioration toward the diabetic range. The sooner habits improve, the quicker biological momentum stalls.

Rebuilding Sensitivity

In the early phases, cell receptors remain capable of re-sensitizing to insulin given the right lifestyle inputs. Early change maximizes that residual metabolic flexibility.

Future Complication Prevention

Keeping blood vessels, nerves, eyes and organs functioning in non-diabetic modes for longer durations pays preventative health dividends for decades down the road.

Psychology Benefits

Perceiving time and control to deliberately halt progression fosters empowerment. Once full diabetes develops, significant lifestyle changes still help, but can feel more daunting. Move urgency from panic toward motivation!

Personalization Options

Subtly abnormal lab results and symptoms provide clues about unique metabolic dysfunction patterns to target before relative deficiencies become absolute. Early customization optimizes results!

The takeaway here is that while prediabetes represents a fork in the road toward illness, another path remains fully accessible with consistent lifestyle tweaks leveraging residual physiological potential. Where you start is not where you'll necessarily finish!

Specific Tactics to Reverse Prediabetes Trajectory

The fantastic news is that preventing full-blown type 2 diabetes even with early biomarkers trending the wrong direction remains largely within your control. Nutrition and lifestyle adjustments profoundly influence how readily cells respond to insulin and process glucose from your bloodstream. Follow these evidence-backed strategies for reversing momentum before it's too late:

Adopt Low Glycemic Eating: Focus on foods minimizing blood sugar spikes and drops that exacerbate insulin resistance over time. Emphasize plants, healthy fats and clean proteins with fiber. Time carbs for after activity.

Fast Strategically: Periodic 12-16 hour gentle fasts allow insulin levels to fully drop and restore receptor sensitivity, especially when combined with resistance training.

Hydrate & Detoxify: Drink adequate water and herbal tea to flush toxins while allowing kidneys to properly regulate minerals influencing glucose metabolism.

Move Daily: Walking just 30 minutes daily helps muscles absorb blood sugar for energy rather than leaving excess glucose in circulation. Mix in strength training and intervals too.

Sleep 7-9 Hours: Restorative sleep optimizes insulin production and sensitivity all day long. Set tech boundaries and soothing nightly wind-downs.

Manage Stress with Rituals: Unmanaged anxiety hormones signal body to release stored glucose. Try meditation, gratitude journaling and affection.

Track Key Markers: Monitor fasting glucose, HbA1c, triglycerides, waist size and other metrics to quantify reversal efforts long-term.

The beauty lies in starting somewhere, anywhere to build positive momentum. Perfect adherence matters less than small consistent efforts towards metabolic improvement in the face of genetic odds. Progress outpaces perfection!

Chapter 3 Takeaways: Destiny is in Your Hands

As we conclude this prediabetes-focused chapter, I hope you feel empowered rather than scared by trends signaling metabolic dysfunction. Remember, early signs and biomarkers creeping outside ideal ranges serve like warning guideposts on the diabetes highway. They prompt self-correction long before hope disappears.

Here are the key lessons I want you taking away:

1. Subtle symptoms and early lab changes are gifts. View rising glucose, HbA1c or triglycerides as helpful feedback to course correct through nutrition and fitness, not unavoidable fate.

2. Consistency moves mountains. Like compound interest, small daily improvements in diet quality, frequent easy movement, stress relief practices and sleep consistency compound over months into dramatic reversal momentum.

3. Leverage strengths of lifestyle medicine. Diabetes is a lifestyle-influenced disease; prediabetes even more so. Medications only mask root causes - daily habits heal them. Commit to changes you can sustain lifelong.

4. Progress supersedes perfection. Don't let great stand in the way of good enough - it's the first step that counts. Maintain new norms rather than allowing stumbles to derail all efforts.

5. This road has been traveled. Millions have halted prediabetes progression through food as medicine principles and sustainable fitness. You have more control than you realize!

I encourage you to embrace, not brace for the days ahead. Your diagnosis is not a destiny if you take purposeful steps forward each day. Surround yourself with support systems to make this journey easier. You've totally got this! Now onward...

Chapter 4: Shielding Your Long-Term Health

If you or a loved one live with diabetes or struggle with ongoing blood sugar regulation issues, you're likely familiar with common downstream complications ranging from heart disease to vision loss that develop insidiously over time. The daily burden of managing medications, appointments, diet restrictions and emotional ups and downs probably feels draining enough without worrying about future catastrophic risks looming ahead.

The promising news is that while diabetes remains incurable, today's management strategies focused on stabilizing glycemic variability and reducing inflammatory influences can dramatically slash downstream disease likelihood. In fact, UK researchers found that diabetes patients reaching an optimal HbA1c level of 6.5% cut their risk of eye, kidney and nerve disease by over 50% compared to those with poorer control above 10%.

In this chapter, I'll distill clinical research around preventing long-term complications into clear guidance on protecting organs and body systems vulnerable to uncontrolled blood sugar's damage over decades. You'll walk away feeling knowledgeable, hopeful and equipped with specific lifestyle medicine strategies to fortify your health starting now.

Specifically, we'll cover evidence-based prevention approaches defending against:

- Heart attacks and strokes

- Kidney dysfunction

- Vision deterioration

- Circulation loss in extremities

- Depression and cognitive decline

Get ready to learn simple, sustainable methods for dodging devastating diabetes-related health crises down the road through daily nutrition and lifestyle tweaks!

Relationship Between Diabetes and Various Complications

To motivate prevention behaviors shielding long-term wellness, it helps to understand precisely how chronically elevated blood glucose and inflammatory fatty acids directly damage arteries, organs and nerves over years and decades after diagnosis. While genetics and lifestyle factors clearly enable type 2 diabetes development, uncontrolled disease progression conversely launches new health crises down the road.

Here's a simplified overview of how diabetes undermines systems vulnerable to vascular dysfunction:

Cardiovascular Disease - Excess circulating glucose infiltrates artery walls, oxidizing cholesterol into plaque obstructing blood flow. Vessels grow stiffer and inflamed. Heart attacks become more likely over time.

Nephropathy - To filter excess sugar, kidneys must work overtime. Gradually, strain damages nephron structures allowing protein leakage into urine. Kidney failure results without improved glucose metabolism.

Retinopathy - Tiny blood vessels supplying the eyes get damaged from metabolic stress. Oxygen deprivation ultimately impairs vision through fluid leakage, scar tissue and blindness.

Neuropathy - Unmanaged blood sugar slowly destroys nerve endings and diminishes small fiber sensation especially in distal extremities. Numbness, pain and reduced mobility result.

Cognitive Impairment - Just as other organs suffer glycemic variability consequences, brain atrophy and dementia risk increase with insulin resistance duration. Memory centers shrink.

As you can see, stabilizing glucose control and lowering inflammation provides tremendous protective effects for delicate body systems under metabolic duress from diabetes. The best defense remains strategically managing root causes!

Protecting Your Heart, Blood Vessels, Eyes, Kidneys and Nerves

While diabetes management often focuses heavily on short-term blood sugar control, making lifestyle choices shielding vulnerable organs and systems from long-term damage matters tremendously for longevity and quality of life. Though medications play a role, research confirms targeted nutrition and fitness adjustments also substantially defend delicate tissues against vascular threats.

Follow these daily strategies protecting what diabetes strains most:

Cardiovascular Defense - Walk 30+ minutes briskly lowering blood pressure, BMI and inflammation while raising protective HDL. Emphasize heart-healthy fats from nuts, seeds and avocado lowering oxidized LDL circulating.

Renal Protection - Stay hydrated with 80+ daily ounces water flushing kidneys and minimizing blood vessel damage. Moderate protein intake avoiding excess waste filtration burden. Choose plant over meat sources.

Vision Vigilance - Boost intake of fruits and vegetables delivering antioxidants, vitamins and minerals nourishing eyes and small vessels especially berries and leafy greens. Support healthy fats and cut sugar.

Nerve Nourishment - Ensure diet includes nervonic acid from cold water fish repairing myelin nerve sheath deterioration over time. Take B-complex helping neurotransmitter function.

Cognitive Clarity - Adopt Mediterranean eating emphasizing brain-boosting healthy fats and polyphenols lowering dementia risk factors. Challenge mind with new skills and social engagement.

While some tissue damage accrues over decades, dedicating daily efforts toward purposeful lifestyle medicine and preventative health behaviors pays tremendous dividends extending vitality years down the road!

Living Well Through Ongoing Management of Biomarkers

As much as total prevention represents an ideal goal, the reality is that some degree of diabetes-influenced organ damage and bodily deterioration inevitable occurs in patients over decades. However, strategic tracking and management of key blood markers and screening tests allows for modulation of risk factors through personalized lifestyle and nutrition adjustments before catastrophic downstream crises arise.

I guide patients on honing daily habits targeting these essential biomarkers:

Hemoglobin A1c - Measures average blood glucose over a 3 month period. Below 7% helps prevent eye, nerve and kidney complications. Address spikes with diet tweaks if creeping up.

Triglycerides - Elevated levels indicate insulin resistance progression and inform treatment paths. Lose weight, cut sugar/alcohol and boost activity to lower.

Kidney Function - Monitor creatinine levels and estimated glomerular filtration rate (eGFR) catching early kidney performance issues tied to vascular health. Stay hydrated and moderate animal proteins.

Cholesterol Panel - Optimizing HDL while lowering LDL and triglyceride ratios through Mediterranean eating and exercise keeps arteries flexible and inflammation controlled.

Blood Pressure - Ideal readings below 120/80mm Hg reduce stroke, cardiovascular disease and cognitive decline likelihood as small vessels remain protected.

While some changes feel outside control, consistently improving daily lifestyle inputs creates significant influence over clinical biomarkers, symptoms, and ultimately, destiny. Disease progression unravels slowly, as does prevention through healthy routines compounding over years.

Chapter 4 Takeaways: Where There's Life, There's Hope

As we wrap up this final chapter focused on sustaining health despite living with diabetes or prediabetes, I want to reiterate this core message: Where there is life, hope abounds. Regardless of what chapter you find yourself in personally, committing to consistent lifestyle medicine for damage control and risk reduction remains well within reach to profoundly influence destinies.

I hope you walk away from this book feeling empowered by these key lessons:

1. Prevention is parallel to treatment. Helping the body heal from the inside out through nourishment, movement and stress relief complements medications managing acute symptoms. Meet your body where it's at through personalization.

2. Shift fixed mindsets. Despite preconceived notions about inevitability of decline, growing research shows that biological trajectories dynamically respond to diet, activity, sleep and environmental inputs defying such fatalism.

3. Celebrate small daily wins. No victory is too minor on this lifelong journey. Milestones like 5 minutes of walking, a vegetable side at dinner, saying no to an extra dessert or taking time to meditate all matter, especially compounded over months and years.

4. You have more power than you may feel. Even amidst diagnosis, genetic odds and progression markers, daily lifestyle inputs profoundly direct the quality and longevity of your vitality timeline, not foretold fate. Recognize and own that influence.

May this book leave you feeling seen, informed, hopeful and equipped with practical, sustainable tools to wield the power you have creating the health destiny made possible by advances in lifestyle medicine. Now go live life vibrantly starting today!

Conclusion: Now Go Defend Your Destiny!

We've covered a lot of ground together in this diabetes lifestyle defense guide - from decoding genetic risk, to outsmarting prediabetes, shielding long term health and everything in between. My deepest hope is that you now feel wholly informed, equipped and empowered to implement personalized prevention and management strategies that allow you to fulfill the vibrant potential within your genetic possibilities.

You may not be able to control susceptibility factors imparted at birth or diagnosis dilemmas nature has dealt you. However, what I want instilled is a sense of RENEWED agency regarding your incredible influence over daily choices - everything from nourishment, movement, sleep, stress relief and so much more - that truly direct diabetes likelihood and lifespan horizons from this day forward regardless of what came before.

Key Takeaways

Let's recap quick high-level highlights to anchor your biggest aha moments into actionable change moving ahead:

Blood Sugar Stability is in Your Hands - Diabetes progresses over years and even decades before thresholds are met. Through food as medicine, activity tweaks, weight management, rest and community, you can profoundly influence hormonal pathways directing your metabolic health destiny in a positive direction at ANY point along that timeline without helplessness. Where attention goes, energy flows!

Lifestyle Overrides Genetic Lottery - Remember, your inherited DNA provides only a predisposition roadmap - whether a smooth highway or rocky trail lies before you depends on the daily navigational choices you make at the steering wheel of sleep consistency, stress reduction, clean eating, movement/play. Suppress risk genes with wise routines!

Progress Beats Perfection - Sustainable change unfolds one small step at a time rather than overnight transformations. As long as your intention stays true to renewed health behaviors compounding lifelong, then slip ups become lessons rather than failures knocking you completely off course. Progress outpaces perfection!

Ongoing Resources

Now go positively disrupt health status quos, flip family fates, refute medical prognoses...and prove lifestyle medicine doubters wrong! I'll leave you with a few resources to continue expanding knowledge on reversing insulin resistance and type 2 diabetes:

The Blood Sugar Solution by Dr. Mark Hyman - Outstanding deep dive into remarkable prevention and reversal outcomes achieved through food as medicine protocols addressing root causes rather than masking symptoms

How Not To Die by Dr. Michael Greger - Accessible introduction to nutritional research powering our bodies toward healing and away from inflammatory Standard American Diets silently enabling "diseases of civilization"

Mastering Diabetes Podcast by Cyrus Khambatta, PhD and Robby Barbaro - Wealth of motivating interviews with plant-based doctors and reversal patients succeeding against all odds through dietary protocols addressing insulin resistance

Final Words: Go Live Vibrantly Now!

Armed with this diabetes lifestyle defense playbook equipping you to proactively support innate self-healing capacities encoded within every cell, organ and system, here begins the first day of genuinely thriving according to your human potential free from metabolic constraint or genetic limitation narratives. Go seize quality longevity starting this very minute. Breathtaking vitality waits for no one - so get busy living brilliantly! Now close this book, lace up some movement shoes or chop veggies for your next medicinal meal. I'll be rooting you on as you step into your brightest Chapter One guided by empowered action rather than fearful reaction. Our destinies await thanks to information coupled with inspiration...so on your mark, get set, start HEALING!

About the Author

A dedicated Doctor of Naturopathic Medicine and wellness coach, Omolola Habib empowers individuals to seize control of their health. With her practical and holistic approach honed through extensive field experience, she has guided numerous people on the path towards improved well-being.

Omolola, fueled by her unwavering commitment to aid others she focuses on offering practical tips and hacks for addressing genetic predispositions; furthermore, she excels in the management of conditions such as diabetes. "*The Diabetes Defense: Practical Tips and Hacks to Shut Down Your Genetic Risk*"--her book reflects not only a profound expertise but also an acute understanding of actionable strategies combating the effects of diabetes along with related health issues.

Omolola, with her unique blend of medical knowledge and wellness coaching: she has made a significant impact on her clients' lives. Under the guidance--and through the support provided by Omolola; individuals have generated meaningful lifestyle changes leading to enhanced health as well as overall well-being.

Omolola, a staunch advocate for holistic health, places unwavering belief in the transformative power of lifestyle medicine. Her clients trust her due to both her compassionate approach and dedicated service; this has established her as an invaluable resource within the realm of naturopathic medicine and wellness coaching.